THE FASTING SIMULATION DIET

Smart recipes for your wellness

CARLO ALBERTO BORGOGNA

CARLO ALBERTO BORGOGNA

Index

CARLO ALBERTO BORGOGNA

PREFACE TO THE NEW EDITION

My previous book "The five days fasting simulation" is a recipe book whose goal is to identify a full menu of five days, for each season of the year, combining the ingredients available in every season, the typical dishes of Italian popular cuisine and the caloric restriction, as disclosed by the most authoritative sources and publications.

With great frankness, I must admit that I never thought I would reach such a large audience with my first book: through several channels, thousands of readers commented on my work in a flattering way and with interesting suggestions.

One of the criticisms that has instead received " The five days fasting simulation" has been related to the complexity of the menus: having to imagine a complete menu, one of the concerns that I considered prior, was the variety of dishes, both to get a mix in line with the guidance of caloric restriction, both to satisfy the sense of satiety.

The goal of my new work is instead practicality: easy, smart recipes and daily menus almost always composed of no more than two or three courses. It will be much easier to manage purchases and preparation and respecting the right proportions of carbohydrates, fats and proteins ... in other words, a recipe book dedicated to those who have a very intense life and do not have time to cook.

The other criticism that has received "The five days fasting simulation" was about the generosity of the portions: in reality, the portions were correctly calibrated, but on the basis of individuals, men and women young and active.

In this new recipe book, an easy-to-understand table allows you to pinpoint your dose with great precision for each recipe.

Finally, for each proposed menu, a complete shopping list is provided: if you have opted for the paper version of the book, the suggestion is to photograph the shopping list with your Smartphone and complete the purchases in a single solution. If you have opted for the digital version, it will be even easier to have the list available even outside the home. In the list you will not find the doses, which are rather strict in the recipes: calibrate the purchase on the largest dose, also because for most of the ingredients you will not be able to buy the amount strictly necessary. Do not forget the frozen foods.

The readers of "The five days fasting simulation" will find in the preface of this book arguments, sources and suggestions already present in the previous publication. The same applies to some dishes similar to those already proposed: please do not consider it a simple repetition, but I suggest you take a cue from the most accurate tables and the simplification of the menus to take advantage of the same benefits in a more practical way.

PREFACE

A recent study conducted by an international team of researchers and published in the scientific journal Cell Metabolism[1] shows that in mature age (up to 65 years) a low protein diet reduces the presence of IGF-1 growth factor, reducing the risk of some types of cancer and in general increases life expectancy.

However, a diet low in protein, especially protein of animal origin, is not for everyone, because it actually means becoming vegetarian and being very parsimonious at the table: for example, who writes is omnivorous, gourmand, wine lover ... without a doctor's prescription, I would never find the motivation to completely change eating habits, giving up some foods that, often, are part of my gastronomic culture. And no ... even for the most willing, it is not enough to practice sports to compensate for the excesses of the table, because it is not (just) to keep fit, it is something more complex than simple weight, directly affects the metabolism.

Other studies[2] show that even a prolonged periodic fasting, if practiced with scientific methods and under medical supervision, allows to obtain considerable benefits, strengthening the immune system and deeply impacting on the metabolism of individuals who practice it

Certainly, however, a prolonged fasting is not for everyone, both because it requires good will, and because it requires health conditions suitable for practicing it, conditions that many do not have.

---

[1] "Low Protein Intake Is Associated with a Major Reduction in IGF-1, Cancer, and Overall Mortality in the 65 and Younger but Not Older Population"; http://www.cell.com/cell-metabolism/fulltext/S1550-4131(14)00062-X .

2 "Prolonged Fasting Reduces IGF-1/PKA to Promote Hematopoietic-Stem-Cell-Based Regeneration and Reverse Immunosuppression"
http://www.cell.com/cell-stem-cell/abstract/S1934-5909(16)00019-9
"A Diet Mimicking Fasting Promotes Regeneration and Reduces Autoimmunity and Multiple Sclerosis Symptoms"
http://www.cell.com/cell-reports/fulltext/S2211-1247(16)30576-9

So is there a method to benefit from the positive effects of these practices, avoiding a lifetime of hardships?

Prof. Valter Longo - Professor of Biogerontology and Director of the Institute of Longevity at USC (University of Southern California) Davis School of Gerontology of Los Angeles and director of the program of Oncology and longevity IFOM in Milan - has formulated a method, the so-called "mima digiuno" or "Fasting Mimicking Diet™". The method allows us to deceive our metabolism: it is a controlled diet for 5 days a month, a quarter or a semester, in which a fasting is simulated, and then returns to normal diet.

The method provides[3] that during the first of five days the caloric intake is reduced by 34% compared to the average needs of the individual, with a distribution of nutritional values of approximately 10% in protein, 56% in fats and 34% in carbohydrates.

From the second to the fifth day, the caloric intake is reduced by 54% compared to the average needs of the individual, with a distribution of nutritional values of about 9% in protein, 44% in fats and 47% in carbohydrates.

The method that simulates fasting is not an isolated event: depending on the subject, the five-day cycle must be repeated several times over the course of a year and possibly for several years.

So how much and what should you eat?

It is not easy to answer this question: being able to put together a five-day vegetarian menu, combining the correct caloric intake and the right balance of nutritional values is very complicated and even more so if you want to respect the seasonality of the

The easiest way is to go directly to L-Nutra[4] a company founded

---

3 https://en.wikipedia.org/wiki/Fast_Mimicking_Diet
http://www.fondazioneveronesi.it/articoli/alimentazione/piu-giovani-e-piu-sani-con-la-dieta-che-mima-il-digiuno

by Prof. Longo, which produces specific dietary foods and programs, which allow a clinical approach to this method, also in support of serious pharmacological therapies.

The other option is to build a complete menu, day by day, perhaps trying to follow the seasonality of food, each with precise doses.

It is from this idea that my first recipe book "The five days fasting simulation" is born and then this my further publication "The fasting simulation diet": a guide containing smart menus that are easy to prepare, to support those who have decided to undertake the fasting simulation diet.

It is very important to specify the following: a low-calorie and low protein diet is a therapy of a medical nature and can only be adopted by healthy adults (WARNING: IT IS INAPPROPRIATE TO CHILDREN) and in any case it should be practiced exclusively on advice and under strict medical supervision. In some subjects, as well as children, just as an example diabetics, this temporary diet could cause serious distress and in the worst case even lead to death.

What you are reading, do not forget, is just a recipe book written by a cooking enthusiast, then

IT DOES NOT BE IN ANY CASE CONSIDERED AS A DIETETIC PRESCRIPTION.

4 http://www.l-nutra.com

QUESTIONS AND ANSWERS

Can I decide by myself to simulate prolonged fasting?

<u>NO.</u>

<u>Fasting simulation or protein / calories restriction has a major impact on your metabolism and can also be very dangerous: you must contact a doctor who must follow you before, during and after.</u>

For those who have intolerances or allergies?

<u>This recipe book does not take into account intolerances or allergies. There are recipes that contain gluten, nuts and other allergens. Check the recipes and evaluate their compatibility with your state of health together with your Doctor: at most you can replace some ingredients with similar ones.</u>

Why should I read this recipe book?

The goal of this recipe book is to identify easy-to-prepare dishes, whose ingredients are compatible with the objectives of caloric and protein restriction in the case of prolonged simulation of fasting.

Four five-days menu proposals are presented in the book.

What are the "forbidden" ingredients?

- No products of animal origin;

- No milk and dairy products;

• No wine, beer and alcohol;

• No sweets and added sugar.

Of course, for those who, like the writer, love wine or beer, it will be a bit more difficult to give up a glass, but remember that it is only five days and that you are following a hypocaloric and low proteins diet that will probably make you feel better for months!

How are the doses calculated?

To each his own: each individual has its own caloric needs that depends on sex, age, height and lifestyle. You can find very interesting information on USDA[5] tables, identifying your profile with a certain precision. However, it must be said that caloric needs are very difficult to calculate with scientific precision: the tables allow us to identify average reference values, which in most of the population are actually realistic.

For each proposed recipe a table is available that allows to determine with a good approximation its own needs, then the restriction objectives: for those subjects that do not fall in the cases reported in the tables, it is however possible to consider the case that is closest , applying a further small correction by excess or default.

Can I use spices?

Spices are allied to this type of diet: they allow to embellish dishes that are often a bit poor by making very few calories: a sachet (or a pinch of stigmas) of saffron is enough to flavor two portions of risotto and the weight is practically irrelevant. The same applies to

---

[5]http://www.cnpp.usda.gov/sites/default/files/usda_food_patterns/EstimatedCalorieNee dsPerDayTable.pdf

turmeric, paprika, chili pepper, oregano, parsley, pepper, etc.

Even the herbs are essential to make dishes more pleasant without impacting significantly with the calories: you will often find in the recipes garlic, chives, parsley, basil, etc.

Can I drink teas and coffee?

Another precious ally are the teas: they have a very minimal caloric intake. But remember not to use sugar and, frankly, I would also avoid using synthetic sweeteners, such as aspartame. If you really cannot do without the sensation of sweet in a tea or an herbal tea, then you can use the Stevia Rebaudiana, which can now be found in sachets ready to use. Remember then that there are mixed herbal teas that provide the use of naturally sweet ingredients, such as licorice or fennel. For the coffee it is very similar: a couple of coffees a day practically have no caloric impact.

Pasta and rice: better whole wheat?

Unless otherwise indicated, both pasta and rice used in recipes are always intended as whole wheat. In particular, for the rice, a semi-processed version is available commercially, which I personally prefer, since it requires cooking times more similar to white rice, but retains many of the nutrients, flavor and part of the brown rice fibers.

When and what to eat?

The menus correspond to the total calories available throughout the day: how to distribute the dishes between breakfast, lunch and dinner is in fact a personal choice, bearing in mind that nutritionists' recommendation is to always prefer breakfast and lunch for the main meal and dinner for a lighter meal. If you have an active life and you are away from home all day, nothing prevents you from eating the main meal in the evening, perhaps avoiding too late and leaving at least three hours from dinner to when you go to bed.

Do I need special cooking tools?

The tool that cannot miss is a precision kitchen scale: you will have to weigh everything, just everything. No other tools are needed that are not already present in every kitchen: pots and pans, oven-proof baking dishes, knives, bowls, cutting boards, a mixer.

How to make the shopping list?

For each five-day menu you will find the relative shopping list. You can buy everything you need at one time, but if you prefer you can buy ingredients day by day. Do not forget the frozen products, which could prove to be a winning card: often the frozen vegetables have excellent quality and they are ready to use, so they will greatly facilitate the cooking.

You will often find in the menu the presence of nuts such as walnuts, hazelnuts, almonds, etc. Also in this case the choice is yours: you can buy fruits still in shell and shell them at the moment or buy bags of nuts ready to use. In any case, keep in mind that the doses refer to the nuts without the shell.

What are the cooking times for rice and pasta?

Cooking times will not be indicated in the recipes. Every pasta size and every type of rice, barley or spelled, have different cooking times that are usually shown on the package by the manufacturer.

Which extra virgin olive oil should I use?

It depends on your preferences.

In Italy, Spain and Greece you can easily find thousands of different types: usually I prefer extra delicate oils for raw foods, for example oils from Liguria Riviera or Garda Lake, while I prefer more tasty oils to season cooked foods, for example oils from Tuscany or Puglia. Up to you, but don't remember that any type of olive oil has exactly the same caloric impact.

It is understood that in the recipes, "olive oil" means "high quality extra virgin olive oil".

CARLO ALBERTO BORGOGNA

DOSES

CARLO ALBERTO BORGOGNA

In the following recipes, you will find a table that allows you to identify, with a certain approximation, the most suitable dose to your physical profile.[6]

What is your physical profile? The table below allows to identify the average energy needs, for males and females, of at least 12 different profiles, considering the three main variables:

- Age: it is considered a single band, adult, between 30 and 60 years;
- Stature: the three most common heights bands are 160 cm, 170 cm and 180 cm;
- Level of physical activity: sedentary, sporty.

Males, between 30 and 60 years:

Profile	Physical activity	Height	Body weight	Average daily energy demand
M1	Sedentary	160 cm	58 kg	2.200 Kcal
M2	Sedentary	170 cm	65 kg	2.350 Kcal
M3	Sedentary	180 cm	73 kg	2.500 Kcal
M4	Sporty	160 cm	58 kg	2.700 Kcal
M5	Sporty	170 cm	65 kg	2.800 Kcal
M6	Sporty	180 cm	73 kg	2.950 Kcal

[6]http://www.cnpp.usda.gov/sites/default/files/usda_food_patterns/EstimatedCalorieNeedsPerDayTable.pdf

Females, between 30 and 60 years:

Profile	Physical activity	Height	Body weight	Average daily energy demand
F1	Sedentary	160 cm	58 kg	1.900 Kcal
F2	Sedentary	170 cm	65 kg	2.000 Kcal
F3	Sedentary	180 cm	73 kg	2.100 Kcal
F4	Sporty	160 cm	58 kg	2.300 Kcal
F5	Sporty	170 cm	65 kg	2.400 Kcal
F6	Sporty	180 cm	73 kg	2.500 Kcal

After identifying the profile that is closest to your characteristics, it will be sufficient to follow, for each recipe, the dose indicated with the relative letter and number.

Samples:

I am male, I am 40 years old, I am 182 cm high, I live very intense days even with walking and I practice at least 3 times a week sport: the profile that comes closest to my features is M6.

I'm a female, I'm 50, I'm 168 cm high, I'm employed in an office and my lifestyle is mainly sedentary: the profile that comes closest to my features is F2.

In the tables of the ingredients, all the doses are indicated in GRAMS.

WARNING: it is very difficult to measure exactly the single portions, therefore, to limit this difficulty at least in part, the doses are always rounded to 5 grams; the only exception is olive oil, which being a 100% fat significantly impacts on the caloric intake, even in the case of rounding a few grams.

In recipes it is often referred to the fine fried mixture: it is a product that is often frozen at the supermarket and is very versatile. Only very minimal doses are sufficient to embellish a dish, so it is never included in the list of ingredients, but sometimes mentioned in recipes. The same applies to all spices, garlic and herbs: they are not mentioned among the ingredients, because they only help to perfume the dishes and have practically no caloric impact: do not miss them in your freezer and in your pantry.

SUGGESTION 1

CARLO ALBERTO BORGOGNA

Shopping list for five days

- Apple
- Asparagus
- Beans
- Bread
- Carrots
- Cherries
- Olive oil
- Flat bread
- Green beans
- Green olives
- Melon
- Nuts
- Onions
- Peas
- Pineapple
- Pistachios
- Potatoes
- Rice
- Short pasta
- Strawberries
- Tomatoes
- Zucchini

Suggestion 1, day 1

The first of the 5 days of caloric restriction, provides a 34% reduced caloric intake compared to the average energy demand.

Rice and peas

Male	*M1*	*M2*	*M3*	*M4*	*M5*	*M6*
Rise	*65*	*70*	*75*	*80*	*85*	*90*
Peas	*150*	*160*	*170*	*180*	*190*	*200*
Olive Oil	*37*	*40*	*42*	*46*	*47*	*50*

Female	*F1*	*F2*	*F3*	*F4*	*F5*	*F6*
Rise	*55*	*60*	*65*	*70*	*75*	*75*
Peas	*130*	*135*	*140*	*155*	*160*	*170*
Olive Oil	*32*	*34*	*36*	*39*	*41*	*42*

Grease a pan with half of the olive oil and toast the rise for a minute on low heat; add the peas and cover with boiling water; salt to taste, add paprika and pepper to taste; when cooked, season with the remaining olive oil

You can leave more or less cooking water, giving rise to the character of a soup or a risotto, respectively.

Pistachios, walnuts and bread

Male	M1	M2	M3	M4	M5	M6
Pistachios	45	45	50	55	55	60
Walnuts	35	40	40	45	45	50
Bread	50	55	60	65	65	70

Female	F1	F2	F3	F4	F5	F6
Pistachios	40	40	45	45	50	50
Walnuts	30	30	35	40	40	45
Bread	45	45	50	55	55	60

You can eat the bread with walnuts and pistachios for breakfast or as a snack during the day.

Apple

Male	M1	M2	M3	M4	M5	M6
Apple	150	160	170	180	190	200

Female	F1	F2	F3	F4	F5	F6
Apple	130	135	140	155	160	170

You can eat the Apple as fruit at the end of the meal or as a snack during the day.

Suggestion 1, day 2

From the second to the fifth day of caloric restriction, a caloric intake of 54% is expected compared to the average energy demand.

Vegetable soup

Male	M1	M2	M3	M4	M5	M6
Carrots	150	160	170	180	190	200
Onions	185	200	210	230	240	250
Potatoes	220	235	250	275	285	300
Peas	150	160	170	180	190	200
Zucchini	150	160	170	180	190	200
Olive Oil	22	24	25	27	28	30

Female	F1	F2	F3	F4	F5	F6
Carrots	130	135	140	155	160	170
Onions	160	170	175	195	200	210
Potatoes	190	200	215	230	245	255
Peas	130	135	140	155	160	170
Zucchini	130	135	140	155	165	170
Olive Oil	19	20	21	23	24	25

Wash and clean the vegetables; cut the carrots, the potatoes, the zucchini and the onions into small cubes; grease a pot with half of the olive oil and cook the onions over low heat for two minutes; add the other vegetables and cover with water; salt to taste and cook for about 30 minutes; at your convenience you can add turmeric, paprika and pepper; at the end of cooking add the remaining olive oil.

Flat bread

Male	M1	M2	M3	M4	M5	M6
Flat bread	60	65	70	75	75	80

Female	F1	F2	F3	F4	F5	F6
Flat bread	50	55	60	60	65	70

You can eat the flat bread to accompany the soup or as a snack during the day.

Cherries

Male	M1	M2	M3	M4	M5	M6
Cherries	185	200	210	230	235	250

Female	F1	F2	F3	F4	F5	F6
Cherries	160	170	175	195	205	210

You can have your cherries for breakfast or as a snack during the day.

Suggestion 1, day 3

From the second to the fifth day of caloric restriction, a caloric intake of 54% is expected compared to the average energy demand.

Green beans salad with potatoes

Male	M1	M2	M3	M4	M5	M6
Green beans	260	280	300	320	330	350
Potatoes	185	200	210	230	240	250
Onions	260	280	300	320	330	350
Tomatoes	225	240	255	275	285	300
Olive Oil	30	32	34	37	38	40

Female	F1	F2	F3	F4	F5	F6
Green beans	225	235	250	275	285	300
Potatoes	160	170	180	195	200	210
Onions	225	235	250	275	285	300
Tomatoes	195	205	215	235	245	255
Olive Oil	26	27	28	31	33	34

Wash and clean the vegetables; steam the green beans, onions and potatoes for 30-35 minutes; cut the diced potatoes and slice the onions and the tomatoes into small slices; arrange all the vegetables in a trigger, salt to taste and season with the olive oil; if you want, you can perfume the salad by adding a peeled garlic clove a few minutes before consuming it (the garlic must be removed).

You can eat still warm or in a salad.

Breadsticks and olives

Male	M1	M2	M3	M4	M5	M6
Breadsticks	60	65	70	75	75	80
Olives	35	40	40	45	45	50

Female	F1	F2	F3	F4	F5	F6
Breadsticks	50	55	55	60	65	70
Olives	30	35	35	40	40	45

You can eat olives with breadsticks as a snack during the day.

Melon

Male	M1	M2	M3	M4	M5	M6
Melon	225	240	255	275	285	300

Female	F1	F2	F3	F4	F5	F6
Melon	195	205	215	235	245	255

You can eat the melon for breakfast.

Suggestion 1, day 4

From the second to the fifth day of caloric restriction, a caloric intake of 54% is expected compared to the average energy requirement.

Risotto with tomatoes

Male	M1	M2	M3	M4	M5	M6
Rise	90	95	100	110	115	120
Tomatoes	35	40	40	45	45	50
Olive Oil	17	20	20	22	22	24

Female	F1	F2	F3	F4	F5	F6
Rise	75	80	85	95	95	100
Tomatoes	30	35	35	40	40	45
Olive Oil	15	16	17	18	19	20

Grease a pan with half of the olive oil and toast the rise over medium heat for a minute; add boiling and salted water; add the past tomatoes sauce; at the end of cooking, add paprika, chili pepper or oregano as you like; serve in a deep dish and season with the remaining olive oil.

Boiled asparagus

Male	M1	M2	M3	M4	M5	M6
Asparagus	225	240	255	275	285	300
Olive Oil	20	20	22	24	25	26

Female	F1	F2	F3	F4	F5	F6
Asparagus	195	205	215	235	245	255
Olive Oil	17	18	19	21	22	22

Wash the asparagus and peel them; cook in boiling water for 20 minutes; arrange them in a flat dish, salt to taste and season with olive oil.

Bread and olives

Male		M1	M2	M3	M4	M5	M6
Whole wheat bread		35	40	40	45	45	50
Olives		35	40	40	45	45	50

Female		F1	F2	F3	F4	F5	F6
Whole wheat bread		30	35	35	40	40	45
Olives		30	35	35	40	40	45

You can eat olives with the whole wheat bread as a snack during the day.

Strawberries

Male	M1	M2	M3	M4	M5	M6
Strawberries	225	240	255	275	285	300

Female	F1	F2	F3	F4	F5	F6
Strawberries	195	200	215	235	245	255

You can eat the strawberries for breakfast.

Suggestion 1, day 5

From the second to the fifth day of caloric restriction, a caloric intake of 54% is expected compared to the average energy demand.

Pasta with beans

Male	M1	M2	M3	M4	M5	M6
Pasta	90	95	105	110	115	120
Beans	115	120	125	135	140	150
Olive Oil	30	32	34	37	38	40

Female	F1	F2	F3	F4	F5	F6
Pasta	75	80	85	90	95	100
Beans	95	100	105	110	120	125
Olive Oil	26	27	28	31	33	34

Cook the beans steamed for about an hour; grease a pot with half of the olive oil, add a teaspoon of fine mixture for sauté and cook over a low heat for a minute; add the beans, water up to cover the beans and salt to taste; after about 15 minutes add the pasta; cook for another 15 minutes and at the end of cooking, add pepper, paprika or turmeric as desired. Serve in a deep dish and season with the remaining olive oil.

NB If the beans are fresh or frozen, steaming will not be necessary; you can go directly to the cooking in the pot, taking care to cook the beans for 30 minutes before adding the pasta.

Pistachios

Male	M1	M2	M3	M4	M5	M6
Pistachios	35	40	40	45	45	50

Female	F1	F2	F3	F4	F5	F6
Pistachios	30	35	35	40	40	45

You can eat salted pistachios as a snack throughout the day.

Pineapple

Male	M1	M2	M3	M4	M5	M6
Pineapple	225	240	255	275	285	300

Female	F1	F2	F3	F4	F5	F6
Pineapple	195	205	215	235	245	255

You can eat the pineapple for breakfast.

SUGGESTION 2

Shopping list for five days

- Almonds
- Apricots
- Barley
- Beans
- Breadsticks
- Capers
- Carrots
- Celery
- Grapes
- Hazelnuts
- Olive Oil
- Olives
- Onions
- Pasta
- Peach
- Peanuts
- Peas
- Prunes
- Tomatoes
- Vegetable gardener
- Walnuts
- Water melon
- Zucchini

Suggestion 2, day 1

The first of the 5 days of caloric restriction, provides a 34% reduced caloric intake compared to the average energy demand.

Pasta and peas

Male	*M1*	*M2*	*M3*	*M4*	*M5*	*M6*
Pasta	90	95	100	110	115	120
Peas	260	280	300	320	330	350
Olive Oil	17	15	16	18	19	20
Female	*F1*	*F2*	*F3*	*F4*	*F5*	*F6*
Pasta	75	80	85	95	95	100
Peas	225	235	250	275	285	300
Olive Oil	12	13	14	15	16	17

Grease a pan with half of the olive oil and cook a pinch of a lightly fried mixture for a minute on low heat; add the fresh peas, boiling water to cover the peas, salt to taste and cook for about 20 minutes; add the pasta, preferably short pasta (e.g. Penne or Maccheroni), directly into the pan, if necessary, other boiling water and cook for another 10-12 minutes, until the water is eat; Serve in a deep dish and season with the remaining olive oil.

Boiled zucchini

Male	M1	M2	M3	M4	M5	M6
Zucchini	260	280	295	320	330	350
Olive Oil	20	25	26	28	28	30

Female	F1	F2	F3	F4	F5	F6
Zucchini	225	235	250	275	285	300
Olive Oil	20	21	22	24	25	25

Wash and clean the zucchini; cook them for about 20 minutes; cut them in two from the long side, obtaining "small boats" and place them in a flat plate; salt to taste and season with olive oil.

You can eat the zucchini still warm if you are at home or prepare them in advance and eat later as a salad.

Apricots, walnuts and almonds

Male	M1	M2	M3	M4	M5	M6
Apricots	300	320	340	360	380	400
Walnuts	35	40	40	45	45	50
Almonds	35	40	40	45	45	50

Female	F1	F2	F3	F4	F5	F6
Apricots	260	270	285	310	325	340
Walnuts	30	35	35	40	40	45
Almonds	30	35	35	40	40	45

You can eat apricots, walnuts and almonds for breakfast or as a snack during the day.

Suggestion 2 day 2

From the second to the fifth day of caloric restriction, a caloric intake of 54% is expected compared to the average energy demand.

Barley salad with tomatoes

Male	M1	M2	M3	M4	M5	M6
Barley	75	80	85	90	95	100
Tomatoes	150	160	170	180	190	200
Celery	150	160	170	180	190	200
Olive Oil	22	24	25	27	28	30

Female	F1	F2	F3	F4	F5	F6
Barley	60	65	70	75	80	85
Tomatoes	130	135	140	155	160	170
Celery	130	135	140	155	160	170
Olive Oil	19	20	21	23	24	25

Cook the barley in boiling salted water for about 30 minutes (or follow the instructions on the package); wash and clean the tomatoes, taking care to eliminate the seeds and obtaining small cubes; wash and clean the celery, taking care to remove the external filaments and cut it into small washers; place the barley in a trigger, add the tomatoes, celery and salt to taste; at your leisure you can flavor with a clove of garlic or a pinch of paprika; seasoned with olive oil.

Breadsticks and hazelnuts

Male	M1	M2	M3	M4	M5	M6
Hazelnuts	35	40	40	45	45	50
Breadsticks	30	30	35	35	40	40

Female	F1	F2	F3	F4	F5	F6
Hazelnuts	30	35	35	40	40	45
Breadsticks	25	25	30	30	35	35

You can eat breadsticks and hazelnuts as a snack throughout the day.

Grapes

Male	M1	M2	M3	M4	M5	M6
Grapes	224	239	254	275	285	300

Female	F1	F2	F3	F4	F5	F6
Grapes	193	203	214	234	244	254

You can have the grapes for breakfast.

Suggestion 2, day 3

From the second to the fifth day of caloric restriction, a caloric intake of 54% is expected compared to the average energy demand.

Beans salad with onions

Male	M1	M2	M3	M4	M5	M6
Beans	225	240	255	275	285	300
Onions	185	200	210	230	235	250
Tomatoes	225	240	255	275	285	300
Olive Oil	30	30	35	35	40	40

Female	F1	F2	F3	F4	F5	F6
Beans	190	200	215	235	245	255
Onions	160	170	180	195	205	210
Tomatoes	190	200	215	235	245	255
Olive Oil	26	27	28	31	33	34

Cook the fresh beans for 30-40 minutes; wash and clean the tomatoes taking care to eliminate the seeds and cut them into small pieces; peel the onions and cut into very thin slices; place the beans in a trigger and add tomatoes, onions and salt to taste; at your leisure you can flavor with a clove of garlic; seasoned with olive oil.

Pistachios

Male	M1	M2	M3	M4	M5	M6
Pistachios	35	40	40	45	45	50

Female	F1	F2	F3	F4	F5	F6
Pistachios	30	30	35	40	40	45

You can eat the pistachios as a snack during the day.

Peach

Male	M1	M2	M3	M4	M5	M6
Peach	225	240	255	275	285	300

Female	F1	F2	F3	F4	F5	F6
Peach	195	200	215	235	245	255

You can have peach for breakfast.

Suggestion 2, day 4

From the second to the fifth day of caloric restriction, a caloric intake of 54% is expected compared to the average energy demand.

Carrots salad with breadsticks

Male	M1	M2	M3	M4	M5	M6
Carrots	300	320	340	365	380	400
Capers	30	30	35	35	40	40
Olive Oil	22	24	25	27	28	30
Breadsticks	100	110	120	130	135	140

Female	F1	F2	F3	F4	F5	F6
Carrots	260	270	285	310	325	340
Capers	25	25	25	30	30	35
Olive Oil	19	20	21	23	24	25
Breadsticks	90	95	100	110	115	120

Wash and peel the carrots; slice the julienne using a knife; place the carrots in a trigger, add the pickled capers, salt to taste and stir; season with the olive oil and enjoy the salad with the breadsticks.

Olives

Male	M1	M2	M3	M4	M5	M6
Olives	45	45	50	55	50	60

Female	F1	F2	F3	F4	F5	F6
Olives	40	40	40	45	50	50

You can eat olives as a snack during the day.

Water melon

Male	M1	M2	M3	M4	M5	M6
Water melon	300	320	340	365	380	400

Female	F1	F2	F3	F4	F5	F6
Water melon	260	270	285	310	325	340

You can eat the water melon for breakfast.

Suggestion 2, day 5

From the second to the fifth day of caloric restriction, a caloric intake of 54% is expected compared to the average energy demand.

Rise salad

Male	M1	M2	M3	M4	M5	M6
Rise	90	95	100	110	115	120
Vegetable gardener	115	120	125	135	140	150
Olive Oil	22	24	25	27	28	30

Female	F1	F2	F3	F4	F5	F6
Rise	75	80	85	90	95	100
Vegetable gardener	100	105	110	115	120	125
Olive Oil	19	20	21	23	24	25

Cook the laugh in boiling water; drain it and place it in a trigger; add the vegetable gardener light, salt to taste and add turmeric, curry or paprika to your liking; season with olive oil.

Peanuts

Male	M1	M2	M3	M4	M5	M6
Peanuts	50	55	60	65	65	70

Female	F1	F2	F3	F4	F5	F6
Peanuts	40	45	50	55	55	60

You can eat peanuts as a snack during the day.

Prunes

Male	M1	M2	M3	M4	M5	M6
Prunes	300	320	340	365	380	400

Female	F1	F2	F3	F4	F5	F6
Prunes	260	270	285	310	325	340

You can eat the prunes for breakfast.

Suggestion 3

Shopping list for five days

- Beans
- Bread
- Breadsticks
- Broccoli
- Carrots
- Crackers
- Green beans
- Hazelnuts
- Leek
- Lettuce
- Olive oil
- Olives
- Onions
- Peas
- Penne pasta
- Pistachios
- *Potatoes*
- Pumpkin
- Tomatoes
- Walnuts
- Zucchini

Suggestion 3, day 1

The first of the 5 days of caloric restriction, provides a 34% reduced caloric intake compared to the average energy demand.

Pumpkin soup

Male	M1	M2	M3	M4	M5	M6
Pumpkin	220	240	250	275	285	300
Potatoes	185	200	210	230	240	250
Leek	150	160	170	180	190	200
Olive Oil	22	24	25	27	28	30

Female	F1	F2	F3	F4	F5	F6
Pumpkin	190	200	215	230	240	250
Potatoes	160	170	180	190	200	210
Leek	130	135	140	150	160	170
Olive Oil	19	20	21	23	24	25

Wash and cut leek into small slices; grease a pan and cook the leek over a low heat with half of the olive oil for two minutes; in the meantime peel the potatoes and the pumpkin and cut them coarsely into cubes; add them to the pan with salt to taste and some water.

After about 15 minutes of cooking, withdraw from the heat; using an immersion mixer, mix everything until a thick cream is obtained; pour the cream into a deep dish and add a pinch of pepper; season with the remaining part of the olive oil.

Breadsticks and walnuts

Male	*M1*	*M2*	*M3*	*M4*	*M5*	*M6*
Walnuts	*75*	*80*	*85*	*90*	*95*	*100*
Breadsticks	*112*	*120*	*125*	*135*	*140*	*150*

Female	*F1*	*F2*	*F3*	*F4*	*F5*	*F6*
Walnuts	*65*	*70*	*70*	*80*	*80*	*85*
Breadsticks	*95*	*100*	*105*	*115*	*120*	*125*

Breadsticks and walnuts is not a recipe, but only a combination that does not require further explanation. You can eat them, for example, for breakfast.

Suggestion 3, day 2

From the second to the fifth day of caloric restriction, a caloric intake of 54% is expected compared to the average energy demand.

Carrots and peas

Male	M1	M2	M3	M4	M5	M6
Carrots	150	160	170	180	190	200
Peas	150	160	170	180	190	200
Onions	75	80	85	90	95	100
Olive Oil	19	20	21	23	24	25

Female	F1	F2	F3	F4	F5	F6
Carrots	130	135	140	155	165	170
Peas	130	135	140	155	165	170
Onions	60	65	70	75	80	85
Olive Oil	16	17	18	19	20	21

Wash and peel the carrots, then cut into small cubes; peel the onions and chop finely; grease a pan with half of the olive oil and cook the onions over a low heat for two minutes; add carrots and peas; add some water, salt to taste and cook for about 30 minutes or until carrots and peas are ready; if you want you can add a pinch of turmeric and paprika; serve in a deep dish and season with the remaining part of the olive oil.

Olives and crackers

Male	M1	M2	M3	M4	M5	M6
Olives	60	65	70	75	80	85
Crackers	50	55	60	65	70	75

Female	F1	F2	F3	F4	F5	F6
Olives	50	55	55	60	65	68
Crackers	45	47	50	55	58	60

Olives and crackers is not a recipe, but only a combination that does not require further explanation. You can eat them, for example, for breakfast.

Suggestion 3, day 3

From the second to the fifth day of caloric restriction, a caloric intake of 54% is expected compared to the average energy demand.

Risotto with zucchini

Male	M1	M2	M3	M4	M5	M6
Rise	90	95	100	110	115	120
Zucchini	225	240	255	275	285	300
Onions	35	40	40	45	45	50
Olive Oil	7	8	8	9	9	10

Female	F1	F2	F3	F4	F5	F6
Rise	75	80	85	95	100	105
Zucchini	195	205	215	235	245	255
Onions	30	35	35	40	40	45
Olive Oil	6	7	7	8	8	8

Grease a pan with half of the olive oil and toast the rise over medium heat for a minute; add boiling and salted water; wash the zucchini and cut them into small cylinders; halfway through cooking, add them to the rise; at the end of cooking, add the salt and adjust if you want a pinch of turmeric; serve in a deep dish and season with the remaining olive oil.

Green beans salad with tomatoes

Male	M1	M2	M3	M4	M5	M6
Green beans	185	200	210	230	240	250
Tomatoes	185	200	210	230	240	250
Onions	75	80	85	90	95	100
Olive Oil	15	16	17	18	19	20

Female	F1	F2	F3	F4	F5	F6
Green beans	160	170	180	195	205	210
Tomatoes	160	170	180	195	205	210
Onions	65	70	70	80	80	85
Olive Oil	13	14	14	16	16	17

Steam the green beans and the onions for about 20 minutes; place in a bowl and let it cool for a few minutes; wash the sliced tomatoes and remove the seeds; add the tomatoes in the bowl and salt to taste, paprika and olive oil; serve still warm.

Pistachios

Male	M1	M2	M3	M4	M5	M6
Pistachios	35	40	40	45	45	50

Female	F1	F2	F3	F4	F5	F6
Pistachios	30	35	35	40	40	45

You can eat the pistachios for breakfast or during the day for a quick snack.

Suggestion 3, day 4

From the second to the fifth day of caloric restriction, a caloric intake of 54% is expected compared to the average energy demand.

Pasta with broccoli

Male	M1	M2	M3	M4	M5	M6
Penne pasta	90	95	100	110	115	120
Broccoli	75	80	85	90	95	100
Olive Oil	11	12	13	14	14	15

Female	F1	F2	F3	F4	F5	F6
Penne pasta	75	80	85	95	100	105
Broccoli	60	65	70	75	80	85
Olive Oil	10	10	11	12	12	13

Cook the pasta penne in boiling salted water; in the meantime wash the broccoli and cook them for about 15 minutes; grease a pan with the olive oil and sauté the broccoli over medium heat for about 5 minutes; drain the pasta pens, add them to the broccoli and adjust the salt; serve in a deep dish.

Green salad with walnuts

Male	M1	M2	M3	M4	M5	M6
Lettuce	75	80	85	90	95	100
Walnuts	20	20	25	25	30	30
Olive Oil	11	12	13	14	14	15

Female	F1	F2	F3	F4	F5	F6
Lettuce	60	65	70	75	80	85
Walnuts	20	20	20	25	25	25
Olive Oil	10	10	11	12	12	13

Wash the lettuce (or use a ready-to-use envelope) and place it in a bowl; coarsely chopped walnuts and add them to the lettuce; salt to taste and season with olive oil.

Breadsticks

Male	M1	M2	M3	M4	M5	M6
Breadsticks	30	30	35	35	40	40

Female	F1	F2	F3	F4	F5	F6
Breadsticks	25	25	30	30	35	35

You can eat breadsticks for breakfast or as a snack during the day.

Suggestion 3, day 5

From the second to the fifth day of caloric restriction, a caloric intake of 54% is expected compared to the average energy demand.

Beans and potatoes

Male	M1	M2	M3	M4	M5	M6
Beans	120	125	135	145	150	160
Potatoes	225	240	255	275	285	300
Tomatoes	90	95	100	110	115	120
Olive Oil	25	25	30	30	35	35

Female	F1	F2	F3	F4	F5	F6
Beans	100	105	115	125	130	135
Potatoes	190	200	215	235	245	255
Tomatoes	75	80	85	95	95	100
Olive Oil	20	25	25	25	30	30

Cook the fresh beans for about 30 minutes; wash, peel and cut the diced potatoes; grease a pan with the olive oil and cook the potatoes for a couple of minutes; add the beans and the tomatoes sauce; cook for about 20 minutes; salt to taste, add a pinch of paprika and serve in a deep dish.

Bread and hazelnuts

Male	M1	M2	M3	M4	M5	M6
Bread	45	45	50	55	50	60
Hazelnuts	20	25	25	25	30	30

Female	F1	F2	F3	F4	F5	F6
Bread	40	40	45	45	50	50
Hazelnuts	20	20	20	25	25	25

You can eat the bread with hazelnuts for breakfast or as a snack during the day.

Orange

Male	M1	M2	M3	M4	M5	M6
Orange	150	160	170	180	190	200

Female	F1	F2	F3	F4	F5	F6
Orange	130	135	140	155	160	170

You can eat the orange for breakfast or as a snack during the day.

SUGGESTION 4

CARLO ALBERTO BORGOGNA

Shopping list for five days

- Apple
- Artichokes
- Chard
- Bread
- Breadsticks
- Cabbage
- Chickpeas
- Crackers
- Grapes
- Hazelnuts
- Leek
- Mushrooms
- Olive Oil
- Olives
- Onions
- Orange
- Pasta
- Pear
- potatoes
- Rise
- Walnuts

Suggestion 4, day 1

The first of the 5 days of caloric restriction, provides a 34% reduced caloric intake compared to the average energy demand.

Risotto with leek

Male	M1	M2	M3	M4	M5	M6
Rise	90	95	100	110	115	120
Leek	150	160	170	180	190	200
Olive Oil	20	21	22	24	25	27

Female	F1	F2	F3	F4	F5	F6
Rise	75	80	85	95	95	100
Leek	130	135	140	155	160	170
Olive Oil	18	19	20	22	23	24

Wash the leek, slice them into thin slices and steam for about 15 minutes; grease a pan on half of the olive oil, cook a pinch of thin fried mixture for two minutes over low heat and add the rise; toast for a minute and add the leek; add boiling water, salt to taste and cook for about 20 minutes; you can add a pinch of nutmeg; serve in a deep dish and season with the remaining olive oil.

Chard

Male	M1	M2	M3	M4	M5	M6
Chard	150	160	170	180	190	200
Olive Oil	17	19	20	22	22	23

Female	F1	F2	F3	F4	F5	F6
Chard	130	135	140	155	160	170
Olive Oil	14	15	16	17	18	18

Wash and clean the chard and cook for about 15 minutes; grease a pan with half of the olive oil and cook a pinch of sauté for two minutes over low heat; add the chard, salt to taste and cook for 10 minutes over low heat; if necessary add some water during cooking; at will you can add a clove of garlic; serve in a deep dish and season with the remaining olive oil.

Hazelnuts, walnuts e crackers

Male	M1	M2	M3	M4	M5	M6
Hazelnuts	30	30	35	35	40	40
Walnuts	30	30	35	35	40	40
Crackers	75	80	85	90	95	100

Female	F1	F2	F3	F4	F5	F6
Hazelnuts	25	25	30	30	35	35
Walnuts	25	25	30	30	35	35
Crackers	65	65	70	75	80	85

You can eat walnuts, hazelnuts and crackers for breakfast or during the day.

Suggestion 4, day 2

From the second to the fifth day of caloric restriction, a caloric intake of 54% is expected compared to the average energy demand.

Spaghetti garlic, oil and chili pepper

Male	*M1*	*M2*	*M3*	*M4*	*M5*	*M6*
Pasta	95	105	110	120	125	130
Olive Oil	15	16	17	18	19	20

Female	*F1*	*F2*	*F3*	*F4*	*F5*	*F6*
Pasta	85	90	95	100	105	110
Olive Oil	32	34	36	39	41	42

Cook the pasta in boiling water; in the meantime, grease a pan with half of the olive oil and cook a clove of garlic and two chili peppers over very low heat; when the pasta is ready, add it to the pan and sauté for a couple of minutes; season with the remaining olive oil.

Cabbage

Male	M1	M2	M3	M4	M5	M6
Cabbage	261	279	297	320	332	350
Olive Oil	10	11	12	14	14	15

Female	F1	F2	F3	F4	F5	F6
Cabbage	225	237	249	273	285	297
Olive Oil	14	15	16	17	18	18

Wash and clean the cabbage and cut it into very thin slices; grease a pan with half of the olive oil and add the cabbage; salt to taste, add a pinch of nutmeg and cook over low heat for about 30 minutes, if necessary add some water; serve in a deep dish and season with the remaining olive oil.

Chickpeas salad with olives

Male	M1	M2	M3	M4	M5	M6
Olives	45	45	50	55	55	60
Chickpeas	150	160	170	185	190	200
Olive Oil	12	13	13	14	14	15

Female	F1	F2	F3	F4	F5	F6
Olives	40	40	45	45	50	50
Chickpeas	130	135	140	155	165	170
Olive Oil	32	34	36	39	41	42

You can use chickpeas in can; put them in a trigger, add the pitted olives and add to the minced parsley or chopped chives; salt to taste and season with olive oil.

Pear

Male	M1	M2	M3	M4	M5	M6
Pear	260	280	300	320	330	350

Female	F1	F2	F3	F4	F5	F6
Pear	225	235	250	275	285	300

You can eat pear for breakfast.

Suggestion 4, day 3

From the second to the fifth day of caloric restriction, a caloric intake of 54% is expected compared to the average energy demand.

potatoes with leek

Male	M1	M2	M3	M4	M5	M6
Potatoes	225	240	255	275	285	300
Leek	150	160	170	180	190	200
Olive Oil	22	24	25	27	28	30

Female	F1	F2	F3	F4	F5	F6
Potatoes	195	200	215	235	245	255
Leek	130	135	140	155	160	170
Olive Oil	19	20	21	23	24	25

Wash and peel the potatoes; wash and cleanse the leek; cook both steamed for about 30 minutes; grease a pan with half of the Olive Oil and cook the leek over a low heat for about 2 minutes; add the potatoes and cook for another 10 or 15 minutes, if necessary add some water; salt to taste and add some chopped chives or chopped parsley; serve in a flat dish and season with the remaining half of the olive oil.

NB If the cooking has not been enough to pulp the potatoes and leek, you can crush them with a fork, until obtaining a viscous consistency, like a coarse mashed potatoes.

Walnuts e breadsticks

Male	M1	M2	M3	M4	M5	M6
Walnuts	30	30	35	35	40	40
Breadsticks	65	70	75	80	85	90

Female	F1	F2	F3	F4	F5	F6
Walnuts	25	25	30	30	35	35
Breadsticks	55	60	65	70	75	75

You can eat the walnuts with breadsticks as a snack during the day.

Orange

Male	M1	M2	M3	M4	M5	M6
Orange	185	200	210	230	235	250

Female	F1	F2	F3	F4	F5	F6
Orange	160	170	180	195	200	210

You can eat the orange for breakfast.

Suggestion 4, day 4

From the second to the fifth day of caloric restriction, a caloric intake of 54% is expected compared to the average energy demand.

Pasta with mushrooms

Male	M1	M2	M3	M4	M5	M6
Pasta	90	95	100	110	115	120
Mushrooms	150	160	170	180	190	200
Onions	150	160	170	180	190	200
Olive Oil	34	36	38	41	43	45

Female	F1	F2	F3	F4	F5	F6
Pasta	75	80	85	95	95	100
Mushrooms	130	135	140	155	160	170
Onions	130	135	140	155	160	170
Olive Oil	29	31	32	35	37	38

Peel the onions and chop finely; grease a pan with half of the olive oil and cook the onions over low heat for about 2 minutes; wash and cut the mushrooms into small cubes and add it to the pan; salt to taste and a pinch of pepper or paprika at your convenience; in the meantime cook the pasta in boiling water; drain the pasta a minute before and add it to the mushrooms in the pan with some cooking water; let the water eat and serve in the bottom dish; season with the remaining half of the olive oil.

Olive and whole grain bread

Male	M1	M2	M3	M4	M5	M6
Olive	50	55	60	65	65	70
Bread	45	45	50	55	55	60

Female	F1	F2	F3	F4	F5	F6
Olive	45	45	50	55	55	60
Bread	40	44	45	45	50	50

You can eat olives with bread as a snack during the day.

Grapes

Male	M1	M2	M3	M4	M5	M6
Grapes	225	240	255	275	285	300

Female	F1	F2	F3	F4	F5	F6
Grapes	195	205	215	235	245	255

You can eat the grapes for breakfast.

Suggestion 4, day 5

From the second to the fifth day of caloric restriction, a caloric intake of 54% is expected compared to the average energy demand.

Artichokes andpotatoes

Male	M1	M2	M3	M4	M5	M6
Artichokes	300	320	340	365	380	400
Potatoes	225	240	255	275	285	300
Olive Oil	37	40	42	46	47	50

Female	F1	F2	F3	F4	F5	F6
Artichokes	260	270	285	310	325	340
Potatoes	1930	200	215	235	245	255
Olive Oil	32	34	36	39	41	42

Browse the artichokes taking care to remove the outer leaves, the thorns and the fibrous part located in the center; cut them into small pieces and sauté over a low heat for 3 or 4 minutes in a pan with half of the olive oil; in the meantime, wash and peel the potatoes, cut them into small dice and add them to the artichokes; cook for another 3 or 4 minutes over low heat, salt to taste and add some water; cook for 20 minutes; serve in a deep dish and season with the remaining olive oil.

Breadsticks

Male	M1	M2	M3	M4	M5	M6
Breadsticks	60	65	65	70	75	80

Female	F1	F2	F3	F4	F5	F6
Breadsticks	50	55	55	60	65	70

You can eat the breadsticks as a snack during the day.

Apple

Male	M1	M2	M3	M4	M5	M6
Apple	220	240	250	275	285	300

Female	F1	F2	F3	F4	F5	F6
Apple	190	200	215	235	245	255

You can eat the apple for breakfast.

TABELLA NUTRIZIONALE DEI PRINCIPALI INGREDIENTI[7]

---

[7] You can check easily and for free nutrition facts on many websites, e.g.: https://ndb.nal.usda.gov/ndb/search/list

Description	Quantity (g)	Proteins (g)	Fats (g)	Carbohydrates (g)	Total Kcal (kcal)
Almonds	100	16	51,5	4	542
Apple	100	0,2	0,3	11	45
Apricots	100	0,4	0,1	6,8	28
Artichoke	100	2,7	0,2	2,5	22
Asparagus	100	3,6	0,2	3,3	29
Barley	100	10,4	1,4	70,5	318
Beans	100	6,4	0,6	19,4	104
Breadsticks	100	12,3	13,9	69	433
Broccoli	100	3	0,4	3,1	27
Cabbage	100	2,1	0,1	2,5	19
Carrots	100	1,1	0	7,6	33
Cauliflower	100	3,2	0,2	2,7	25
Chard	100	1,3	0,1	2,8	17
Cherries	100	0,8	0,1	9	38
Chickpeas	100	4,3	1,4	7,2	56
Crackers	100	8,8	17,2	58,1	443
Grapes	100	0,5	0,1	15,6	61
Green beans	100	2,1	0,1	2,4	17
Hazelnuts	100	13	62,9	1,8	625
Leek	100	2,1	0,1	5,2	29
Melon	100	0,8	0,2	7,4	33
Mushrooms	100	2,3	0,4	1,9	20
Olive oil	100	0	100	0	900
Olives	100	1,6	25,1	0,8	234
Onions	100	10,2	1,7	68,6	313
Orange	100	0,7	0,2	7,8	34
Pasta	100	13,4	2,5	66,2	324
Peanuts	100	29	50	8,5	597
Pear	100	0,3	0,4	9,5	41
Peas	100	7	0,2	12,4	76
Pineapple	100	0,5	0	10	40
Pistachios	100	20,6	48,4	14	577
Potatoes	100	2,1	1	18	85
Pumpkin	100	1,1	0,1	3,5	10
Rise	100	6,7	2,8	81,3	357
Strawberries	100	0,9	0,4	5,3	27
Tomatoes	100	1	0,2	3,5	19
Walnuts	100	15,8	63,7	6,3	660
Water melon	100	0,4	0	3,7	15
Whole wheat bread	100	7,5	1,3	53,8	243
Zucchini	100	1,3	0,1	1,4	11

CARLO ALBERTO BORGOGNA

BIOGRAPHY OF THE AUTHOR

CARLO ALBERTO BORGOGNA IS A GENERAL MANAGER WITH AN INNATE PASSION FOR THE KITCHEN. LOVER OF WINE IS A PASSIONATE FOLLOWER OF SLOW FOOD FROM THE VERY BEGINNING OF THE ASSOCIATION. HE IS INTERESTED IN FOOD, WELLNESS, ENVIRONMENTAL SUSTAINABILITY, BUT ITS MAIN ACTIVITY IS THAT OF DAD.

Made in the USA
Las Vegas, NV
10 December 2020